Copyright **2018** by Jodi Rose

Inmate Support /Incarcerated LO's
Like us on Facebook-

Inmate Support

Presents

"FUELED"

An Insider's Guide to Transforming the Mind, Body, and Soul for the Incarcerated Man.

Compiled by Jodi Rose

Written by "Big Steve" Incarcerated in Texas Department of Criminal Justice

<u>**About the Author**</u>

Big Steve's Workout Corner

Hey fellas, my name is Chris aka Big Steve, Here's a little bit of background on myself.

I got put on probation for burglary of a habitation when I was 17, my sentence was 7 years deferred probation. During that time, I struggled with drugs and alcohol until I gave up the drug life and traded it in for the gym life when I was 20. I dedicated myself to health and fitness absorbing all the information I could get my hands on. I became a personal trainer through the American Council on Exercise with my eyes set on eventually achieving a doctorate in kinesiology to become a physical therapist with the long term goal of teaching kinesiology to college students.

Well my plans got put on pause halfway through my Bachelor of Art degree when I revoked my probation by failing a drug test for alcohol. It was an expensive lesson as it cost me getting sentenced 10 years to prison after completing 6 $\frac{1}{2}$ years of 7 years' probation. I currently have 2 $\frac{1}{2}$ years done and am most likely a short way to the door. I have spent the last few years having to make the best workouts possible with limited resources and I would be honored to share what I've learned with you guys.

Included in this book is information relating to eliminating rep madness, proper cardio habits workout programs using common room fixtures, diet guidelines, and other miscellaneous habits that are important to pick up while being incarcerated.

Some of you will be beginners with a lot of new found time on your hands looking for ways to use it productively. I want to commend you for trying to use your time to develop one of the only meaningful things you can take with you out of prison. For those of you with some experience in the workout game I encourage you to keep an open mind. Nothing kills the progression of knowledge faster than pride getting in the way. I am constantly learning and during my journey I've learned the things I thought I knew were unfounded myths. If at any point you read something in my work you disagree with, I encourage you to do your own research and find the truth for yourself! And no Fellas, Men's Health magazine is not research, a high percentage of articles in those magazines are geared towards selling a product. A pair of lips will tell you anything especially where money is involved so check your sources and don't get duped into bad workout advice. Look for information by people through the NASM (National Association of Sports Medication) or similar research communities.

Now guys I want to close this intro except with my mission statement for this project. "I am writing from my knowledge and experience to help build up inmates in areas of lasting weakness". I am a Christian and my bible says "all things work together for good for those who love God" Romans 8:28. Is a verse that comes to mind, it says: As for you, you meant evil against me but God meant it for good". We've been dealt a tough hand guys. If I had taken what they were originally offering me I would have been out 18 months ago. If that had happened, I most likely would have missed out on the opportunity to apply the principles of dedication and commitment I learned in the fitness word, to the spiritual. I encourage you men, as we go into how to build up your physical bodies, allow these principles of consistent dedication and commitment to over flow into the only other meaningful thing you can take with you, your spirit. 1 Timothy 4:8 says "While bodily training is of some value, Godliness is of value in every other way, as it holds promise for the present life and the life to come". Just like we have physical muscles and appetites, we have spiritual muscles and appetites too. As we make the best physical workouts out of enemy surroundings and feed our muscles with cornbread and commissary I pray that you use this time to allow God to work on your character and to feed your soul with daily time in his Holy word. That being said let's get to the gains!

Section 1

Rep Madness

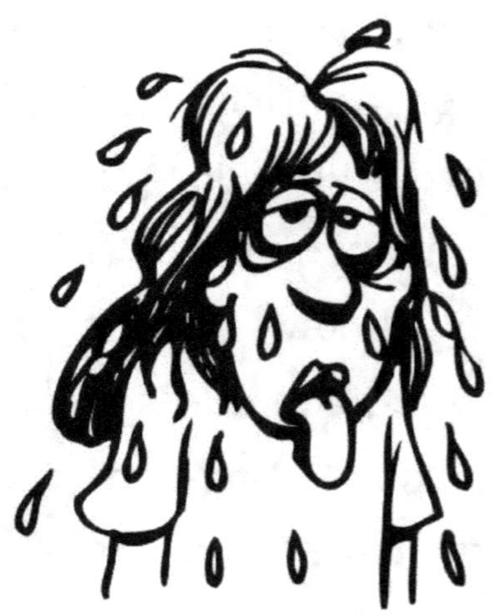

How many of you guys have heard this question? "What did you do for your workout today"? Well we started with 30 down (32 steps starting at 30, 29,28 etc. in descending order) regular pushups, then we did 25 down incline pushups (210), and finished with 20 down decline pushups (120). If you've been adding along with me that's 655 pushups! Some of you may be scoffing right now saying: "Psh I do 1,000 pushups" every other day". Brothers let's stop this madness! Let's get real here any of us really seen any substantial gains behind doing 1000 pushups?

The principle we are going to discuss into practice is how the gains could increase exponentially. Genetics plays a big part in how quick we gain muscle and burn fat. Being convicts we've learned a lot about maximizing the hand we're dealt and there

is no reason not to apply that skill to our
workouts.

When I turned myself into county
with 8 years of gym experience under my
belt I was 230 lbs., 8% body fat, on a 6'
frame. I was doing alright and when my
incarceration started I had very little
experience working out outside of a gym
setting. I joined a 1000 rep work clique and
while my reps were increasing, my weight
was dropping and my body fat was
increasing. I was devastated, my muscle
soreness was unreal. I was starving from
the kid's meals they feed us, I was
watching my gains steadily disappear. I
knew something had to change. Well, fellas
the best answers are usually the simplest
ones. I thought back to the basic principles
of fitness pros like Arnold, Ronnie, and Kai.
Everyone is in agreement that for your
muscles to grow they must be overloaded.
Overloaded means you're demanding more

work from your muscles than they are capable of performing. If you don't tell your muscles that they need to grow, then they won't grow folks, simple as that! How do you tell your muscles they need to grow? By pushing them to the point of failure! Now some of you may be saying "wait a minute Big Steve, I've been hitting failure in my rep regimen, what's the difference? Hitting failure earlier than your 15th rep is overloaded, anything higher than that is simply fatigue. Not only is pushing your muscles to fatigue not helping you reach your optimal level of muscle gain, it can also be counterproductive causing you to also lose gains. This is why, your muscles have stored glucose available for energy, this stored energy source is called glycogen. When your sets are exceeding 15 reps you are depleting your available glycogen and causing muscles to be torn down past the optimal point of protein synthesis and maximum muscular development. I would rather see someone do 5 sets of 5 than do 30 sets of 30 to achieve failure, 4-6 reps are the optimal for strength, 6-12 is optimal for hypertrophy. We need to work smart to achieve the gains fellas.

So how do we achieve failure in less than 15 reps you ask? We need resistance, this is why a good workout partner is critical. With a good work out partner you can achieve resistance by him pressing or standing on your back as you progress in your push up game. He can hold a towel to give you resistance on your bicep game. This resistance to achieve failure before your 15th rep every set is crucial guys. If you don't push yourself to over load, not fatigue, not exhaustion, but overload 95% of us will not gain without it. Stop the rep madness brothers!

Now I know it can feel like were being pushed further than our spiritual muscles can take us on a daily basis. The weight of incarceration is on our shoulders every day. We encounter resistance every day with the boss man talking crazy to us, constantly wondering if that parole is coming soon, and the list goes on infinitely. Sometimes we wonder if we have the strength to go on. Let me assure you that God is familiar with the principle of over load. In 1 Corinthians 10:30 it says "God is faithful and he will not let you be tempted beyond your ability, but with the temptation he will also provide the way of escape, that you may be able to endure it". When we succumb to a temptation God is exposing a weakness in our life. Looking at it from a spiritual perspective God is trying to develop our spiritual muscles by putting that resistance in our life. I came to jail physically strong but spiritually I was a sissy. That temptation would rise up and I would burn off on Gods way out for drugs, fast women, and fast money. The result was where I'm sitting now. There is a reason we're told to "count it all joy my brothers, when you meet trials of various kinds, for you know that the testing of your faith produces steadfastness. Let steadfastness have its full effect that you may be perfect and complete lacking in nothing" in James 1:2. God knows that it takes someone spiritually jacked to consistently choose his way out of temptation instead of our way into prison. Anything worth having in life takes a little bit of sacrifice ya'll. I encourage you to stay focused on your spiritual gains and don't let that resistance get you down. I will end this section with this: when the disciples were in a boat during the storm while Jesus was on the shore, it says in Mark 6:48 "Then he saw them straining and roving, for the wind was against them (kind

of like doing 1000 reps). My point
brothers, is that God sees you. He knows
our struggles; he sees our strain. The story
ends by the Lord calming the storm. It
took later into the 4th watch of the night
but he was faithful. Stop the madness of
uselessly flowing without hope. Use the
storm to grow spiritually but know that God
will quiet that storm.

Section 2

Mindset of Wellness

Mind-sets of wellness

     I would like to start by submitting your consideration to proverbs 23:7. The KJV renders the verse "As a man thinketh so also is he".   King Solomon 3000 years ago was aware that our thoughts define us. Modern medicine has proven that or thoughts are proportionally relational to our health. Anyone with and intermediate experience in with working out can attest to the fact there are some days when your head's not in it. You got enough sleep, you've maintained your diet, and your motivations just not there. What gives? On days like these I've learned from experience that if I can put my discouragement aside and put a gag in the mouth of the negative voice in my head saying "I just don't feel like it today", then I usually end up having one of the most fruitful workouts I've had in a long time. Experiences like these are the reminders I need to keep in the forefront of my mind when the I don't, I want, and "I cants" crop up. As King Solomon said (I'm paraphrasing) it's all in your head, and sooner we can internalize that, the sooner we can begin to overcome our own negativity. As we train and strengthen our bodies most of us will realize we have all along been strengthening our minds simultaneously. After all it takes a certain, special type of mental fortitude to set up 2 hours before your day actually starts to get your workout in. It takes certain type of drive to continue to stay dedicated while you are incarcerated and nobody but you can see your results. It takes a special type of person to try to maintain a healthy diet in a world of starches, spreads, and cakes. You my friend are that type of person! So whenever your mind tries to tell you otherwise, you tell that negative voice to shut its trap and you go out and prove it wrong.

Now of course there are some strategies to help us avoid getting into one of those negative funks but before we discuss them let's take a look at what we can learn from the ancient Greeks. In Greek mythology there is a seductive singing creature called a siren. Well this particular creature lives in a water filled gorge in which boats some time pass through. When a boat passes, the siren starts singing a seductive song that sends the sailor to his death. No one has survived while passing through this canal. Well one Greek hero decides he wants to be the first to hear the sirens song and live. So, he prepares his ship and ready's his crew by putting wax in their ears. He then has them tie him tightly to the mast of the ship and they begin their voyage. When they reach the canyon the song begins and the

bound Greek hero starts fighting against
the bonds eyes bulging and veins protruding
he struggles to squirm against his binding
but they turn and he lives and is the first
to leaves the canyon in one piece. Even
though he survives, for the rest of his life
he is haunted by the sirens serenade.
Another Greek hero, out of necessity,
enters the same canyon. Only this time
when the sirens song starts he grabs his
harp and plays like he's never played
before. The sirens ominous melody is still
audible but it is over powered by the closer
tune of the captain's harp and the whole
crew is enraptured by his passionate
performance. They too make it through the
canyon unharmed. The point here is there
can a be multitude of ways to reach a
destination but the effects of the journey
can be completely different.

　　　If we focus on the intensity of the
work out and get bound up into a stiff

inflexible, never enhancing routine then we might be more apt to surrender to the seductive crying to knock off the path of progress. If our diet is so strict never allowing ourselves to indulge in a tasty treat, we may find ourselves overwhelmed and hoisting a white flag of surrender. If we're constantly dreading the work, we have put in instead of focusing on the gain we can pull out then it's easy to get over whelmed. For these reasons it's important that we keep a check on our attitudes and mind sets.

Now at the beginning of this particular topic I spoke on our heads not being in it when we're well rested and well fed. That was because the surest ways for our thoughts, attitudes, and drive to sour are when we are hungry and tired. If we're encountering a mental road block start by checking those two first. I know in prison it is hard to sleep and we don't get much to eat, but we will talk about ways to work that out as well later in this reading.

The next thing that can hinder our attitudes are boredom. Have we been using exactly the same routine for more than 90 days? Has it been more than 90 days since we took a week off to de-load work? If so, take a break and change it up! Another common pitfall is having low intensity long workouts. For physiological reasons used previously we've outlined why shorter workouts are better, but there is a psychological component as well. Many people can find a long workout tedious with their energy drained way before the workout is over causing a ceiling to be set over the amount of gain. Remember we are looking for quality and not necessarily quantity. There is nothing that kills motivation faster than investing a huge quantity of time in a workout that is yielding low quality gains. It's better to give it your all for a shorter period than feel forced to divulge through a long convoluted routine. You'll get more out of it for a much lower investment premium.

Another thing that can wreck our motivation is when our diet is in disarray. I'm not talking about our 2-3 cheat meals a week; I'm talking about see food diet. You see food and eat it. Obviously eating what we want is going to affect our gains and hinder our positive mind frames. One toxic mind-set is eating junk food and saying "oh, I'll run it off later" or saying "I had to do without today I deserve to eat like trash". The longer you maintain a healthy diet and an active lifestyle the less you will crave the junk. You will begin to want to reward your bodies. I have also heard from others dude's things like "being locked up there is no way to eat healthy". I will show you how that mind set can be turned around because it is false.

Let's try hard work with healthy foods instead of squandering your hard work with a reckless diet. Step out on faith and let that inner transformation begins to change your mind set from "I deserve junk food" to "I deserve to reward my hard work with wholesome food".

Another destructive mind-set is to focus on the pain it takes to get to the gain instead of focusing on the gain itself. Some days I just really don't feel like doing cardio at the appointed time and place. On days like these it's important for me to remember that euphoric feeling of a workout well done. I have to remember the energy boost I get for the rest of the day as a result of an increased metabolic rate. And of course I know those Abs aren't going to define themselves. If I want to stay fit and never sloppy by the time of my release, then I know it's important to focus on the destination and not let the hurdles that trip me up. After all a wise man once told me "Anything worth having in life, you aren't going to get it unless, you give a little bit of sacrifice".

Finally, to exhaust the ancient Greek analogy in the physical realm, let's look at a common denominator between both heroes. They both had companions; they had a crew to see them through to the other side. This is significant because it illustrates how vital having help can be to accomplish our goals. A workout partner is important to help with encouragement and motivation as we discussed previously. Take it a step further though and imagine if you had support beyond that! What if you could encourage your spouse at home to desire to eat healthy and live an active life style? What if you had a group of people at work training together for a sporting event or an obstacle course run or even just a body fat % reduction contest with a prize for the winner? What if your kids are in a soccer league and they love it? All of these ideas and many more can be the difference between life and death in the longevity of your workout program. If you have a positive reason, involving a loved one or friend, to stay dedicated, it will be much easier to stick with it. If you have people surrounding, you keeping you accountable and motivated then the sky is the limit. If a love of good wholesome nutritious food is being cultivated in your home then not only will you and your family's gains come much quicker, but the overall atmosphere of wellness will be conducive to a higher quality of life over all. Who doesn't want that? So don't cram it down anyone's throat but whenever you can encourage those around you to live active healthful lives take advantage of the opportunity. "And let us consider how to stir up one another to love and good works" Hebrews 10:24.

Alright folks lets go ahead and enter into the 4th dimension here because after all having fit physical bodies is important, but even more important is our spiritual fitness. The apostle Paul identified that there is indeed a time to bind when it comes to combatting negative thoughts and attitudes. Let's take a look at one of the single most powerful passages in scripture when it comes to spiritual warfare. It tells us in 2 Corinthians 10:3-5 says "For though we walk in the flesh, we are not waging war according to the flesh but have divine power to destroy stronghold. We destroy arguments and every lofty opinion raised against the knowledge of God, and take every thought captive to obey Christ". Paul tells us to take our thoughts captive. This means that we stop the negative ones from having freedom and liberty in the ships of our minds. It also prevents them from being seduced out of our minds in the forms of actions by the seductive siren songs of temptation that we encounter on a daily basis. James 1:14-15 tells us "Each person is tempted when he is lured and enticed by his own desires then desires when it has conceived gives birth to sin and sin when it is fully grown brings forth death". This passage tells us we all have sinful desires but the sin is <u>born</u> by the acting of these desires. Martin Luther compared thoughts to birds when he said "you can't stop a bird from flying overhead but you can stop him from nesting in your hair" (or beard in my case). You see it is the union of the desire and our human will in actions that conceive sin and there was only one person to ever walk the planet to have a perfect relationship between his desires and his human will have controlled actions. His name is Jesus Christ and the reason the relationship was perfect can be found in John 6:35 "For I have come down from heaven, not to do my own will but the will of him who sent me". Now hold on this Jesus, God in the flesh, why is he not relying on his own will? Because, while fully God he is also fully human. We have evidence in the garden of Gethsemane that Jesus' human desire was contrary to God's will. Matthew 26:39 says "My father, if it be possible let this cup pass from me, nevertheless not as I will but as you will". Jesus knew his human desire to avoid suffering was far inferior to God's master plan. But the fully God side of Jesus' nature allowed and empowered Him to set His own human will aside and submit to the will of God. By Him doing this he opened the door for each one of us to do the same by allowing us to become partakers in the divine nature of God (2 Peter 1:4). Jesus won this spiritual battle because first he had knowledge of

God's will and second because he put his human nature aside to submit to it, becoming an example for all those that follow him.

So let's talk about knowledge. We won't know which thoughts to take captive if we don't know which are "against the knowledge of God" I've encountered many people that claim to know God yet deny the accuracy of the Bible or our ability to get to know Him. How are we supposed to serve Him if we have no idea who He is and what His plan is for us? So many of us have taken God from his position of complete perfection and sovereign authority and regulated him to the equal of a doting grandfather. We may want the occasional gift and wisdom God gives us. We enjoy His presence during the holiday season. But when it comes time to conform to His plan for us how many of us take it seriously? I was like this in the past, but doesn't our creator and sovereign ruler of the universe deserve more than this? Now you may be thinking but Big Steve, God's never dropped a letter in the mail to me outlining his will so how are we supposed to know?" The Bible is a book consisting of 66 books written over a 2500-year period of time by 40 different authors that all agree about the nature of fallen man, the nature of holy sovereign God and his plan of redemption for us. The Bible is our source knowledge of God's will for us and it is our key to overcoming thoughts and desire contrary to the knowledge of God. Hebrews 4:12 says "For the word of God is living and active, sharper than any two-edged sword, piercing to the division of souls and spirit, of joints and marrow, and discerning the thoughts and intentions of the heart". It goes down to the core of our being and separates out corrupt, fleshy, human desires from those of Gods perfect design.

Now how do we turn those words on paper into a razor sharp spiritual weapon? First off you're on the right path because all throughout the Bible God promises to reveal things to those that look for it. "Seek me and you will find me" says the Lord. In the book of Revelation when no one could be found to open the scroll John the beloved disciple fell down and wept. The angel told him to dry his tears and "Behold the Lion of the tribe of Juda can open the scroll". Revelation 5:5. The point is God reveals things to those that seek him. God sees you in your quest to find Him and if you persevere you will be rewarded with that which you seek.

Second we have to put our pride and human wisdom aside. Jesus prayed in Matthew 11:25 "I thank you, Father, Lord of heaven and earth that you have hidden those things from the wise and understanding and revealed them to the little children". Nothing can stand in the way of acquiring knowledge than the assumption that you already have it. We have to grow into our spiritual rebirth as we grew into our physical maturity. God has told us in Isaiah 53:8 my thoughts are not your thoughts neither are your ways my ways. We suffer from a spiritual blindness that Christ has begun the process of restoring. Seeing the world around us with our 5 senses is like looking through a prison (what's up can be down if what's down can be up). Add sin into the mix and our sight perception begins to look like a laser light show at a rave. Flashing lights distorting our view of reality and multi colored lights all for our attention to come and distract us from reality as God sees it. It's important to come to God in the spirit of humanity and open mindlessness allowing him to mold us into His will instead of trying to bundle Him up into our will.

And third is an issue of POWER. 1 Thessalonians 1:5 says "because our gospel came to you not only in word, but also in power and in the Holy Spirit with full conviction". Let's talk about the first occurrence of power being associated with Christ in the flesh. In Luke 11:41, 1:80, 2:40, 2:52, and 4:1 (look them up for yourself) we see Jesus being filled with favor, wisdom, and stature. It isn't until after Jesus is baptized and the Holy Spirit descends upon Him like a dove that spirit drives Him out into the wilderness to overcome the temptations that we hear about power. After Jesus triumphs over the temptations using the word of God we arrive at Luke 4:14 "And Jesus returned in the Power of the Spirit to Galilee", where he began his ministry. How beautiful is that? Even our Lord and Savior had to set the example and resist the temptations, using the word of God, to receive the Power of the Spirit. This is a monumental truth for us in our walk. Once we're saved (justified in the spirit of God) satan is going to do anything to try and steal our power so we can't use it. We must always be prepared to combat satan in his lies and schemes he puts on us.

Section 3

Jailhouse Nutrition

Jail House Nutrition

"Put the honeybun down! "

So this chapter has been a difficult one for me because how "they" feed us can be so far away from what we are supposed to eat that it can "seem" like we are constantly fighting a losing battle. I've wondered if it is even worth including a real world nutrition section, but the way I see it, Lord willing, those doors will open one day and I believe it will be beneficial to go ahead and prepare you for that day as well. Remember we are embarking on a whole new lifestyle of wellness that can't simply end when we touch down. Until that time though, a lot of jail house nutrition tips will be choosing the lesser of two evils, so let's begin.

Alright now I'm thinking at least 99% of us started our incarceration in county jail. For those of you in that phase of your incarceration my heart goes out to you. I did 25 months in county fighting a case myself. I know the struggles you are facing with 3 trays a day well under 2000 calories and commissary prices that can be compared to highway robbery. I'm sure ya'll know how expensive it can be to eat healthy or even just eat enough calories with the very limited selection we have access to. For those of you that are very picky and don't like vegetables, it's time to get over that because you are about to get "vegetable's out the game" I don't want to sound like your mom but on a serious note those vegetables will help you achieve a better fullness and add vitamins and minerals in an already vitamin deficient diet. Plus, vegetables will be a big part of living a healthy lifestyle when you get out so adjusting you taste buds now to the gross ones will get you ready to eat fresh ones upon your release. I hated beans before I came to jail, couldn't stand them! Hunger and a need for as much protein as humanly possible overcame my compunction over beans and now I can't imagine not liking them. Your taste buds can change.

If your goal is to put on muscle, because of the severe lack of nutritious food, you will probably need to eat everything on your trays, consume a high protein post meal, and up your calories by adding a rice/bean/fish type meal on your strength training days. By severe lack of notorious food, I mean foods that are high in calories without providing a proportional number of vitamins, whole grains, and proteins. Examples of these you can expect to see often on your trays are white bread, biscuits, pancakes, mushed potatoes, noodle trays with a teaspoon of meat, cakes, and cookies. These are items with a high calorie count that help the state achieve the minimum net calorie count required by law while at the same time depriving our bodies of the whole grains, complex carbs, and proteins our bodies need to retain good health and fitness. For these reasons consuming the amount of food you need to build muscle, while incarcerated, may cause you to gain some fat at the same time, as the extra calories consumed to meet our protein and carb needs are turned to fat for storage. This is why most body builder's cycle back between bulking and cutting diets. A "dirty bulk", which would be similar to what our muscle gaining diet in jail would be, can add up to a pound of fat for every pound of muscle. This is because we don't currently have access to lean foods and complex carbs our body needs to gain muscle while minimizing fat gains. In the world of "dirty bulk" is usually either due to laziness or because its winter time and the little extra bulk from fat can be concealed under sweaters and hoodies. It is much easier to burn fat than it is to build muscle. That Is another reason many people choose to dirty bulk, because they know that muscle gained can be maintained and the extra fat can be shed 3-6 months down the road when you adjust your diet to burn fat or "cut". This is done by manipulating your "micro-molecule" intake. Every time I refer to micro-molecules I am talking about the distribution of carbohydrates, proteins, and fits in your diet.

Proteins are the building blocks of your muscular tissue. Amino acids are the building blocks of these proteins. When we tear our muscles down through strength training, our bodies use proteins to rebuild that muscular tissue. There are at least 20 different Amino acids that make up protein and 8 – 10 of them are considered essential. Essential Amino Acids are called essential because they cannot be produced by the body and must be consumed by the diet. Incomplete proteins are proteins that are lacking in 1 or more of the essential amino acids, these are considered lower quality proteins. Almost all plant foods are incomplete proteins and will need to combine with complimentary proteins.

This is where vegetarians without proper knowledge of the food they need to combine to make a complete protein can get into trouble. This is also the problem with reading the label on say a packet of oatmeal. Three may be 4 grams of protein in a packet but if that oatmeal isn't combined with some milk, peanut butter, or nuts then you aren't receiving all the amino acids your body needs to make a complete or higher quality protein. Plant and dairy proteins that need to be combined to make complete proteins can be grains and dairy/grains and nuts/ grains and legumes/ milk and legumes/ and nuts and legumes. If you're wondering what a legume is you're not alone, common example are beans and nuts. Try combining those to make the higher quality proteins your body needs. Any animal protein is a complete protein. The only problem with that is that many animal proteins are also high in fat and cholesterol. Lean animal proteins would be fish, chicken, and egg whites. I am currently in prison where they breed their own pigs. We have pork every day. So yes in consuming more much needed grains of protein but at the cost of additional fat and cholesterol. See what I mean about fighting a losing battle? Thankfully most prisons offer mackerel packs give around 80 grams of protein so there are always ways to overcome these obstacles. The question is Simply how far are you willing to go to meet your goals? Another danger commonly encountered while trying to meet your daily need intake is the "peanut butter fat trap" looking at the label we can expect to see something like 7 grams of protein x 16 servings at a price between $1.50 and $5.00 a jar. Now we might be thinking hello best bang for your buck! Meeting that 112 grams of protein in $3.00 and 18 gram of protein tuna packs would cost about 17 bucks. Now on the outside it may appear like we're winning until we examine the ingredients on the peanut butter and take into account what we just learned about incomplete protein. That 7 grams of protein is costing us 16 grams of fat, mostly from partially hydrogenated vegetable oil. Anything partially hydrogenated is the worst kind of fat you can eat aside from trans-fat. Since it is solid at room temperature your body has a very hard time processing it and in addition its chalk full of low-density lipo proteins or LDL's which are known as the bad cholesterol. That is because this type of cholesterol is linked to heart disease and the hardening of the arteries leading to increased risk for stroke. In addition to make that peanut butter a complete protein it needs to be combined with a complimentary vegetable protein.

So as you can see that 12 dollars you're saving at the store window between a $5 jar and 17 dollars of tuna packs will cost you in complimentary proteins and possible medical bills to deal with the plagues build up in your arteries later down the line. Now I don't believe you need to ex the peanut butter completely but, moderation should definitely be practiced with your consumption. I try to make 1 jar last 2 – 3 weeks to avoid over loading myself with all that bad fat and just as all protein isn't create equal neither are all fats created equal.

Saturated fat is fat that is solid at room temperature. This causes it to be static i.e. have a longer shelf life (Hello, commissary window). The other characteristics of a saturated fat is that it contains a high (Bad Cholesterol) content which is a reason to try to avoid saturated fat as much as possible consuming less than 10% of our calories for the day in saturated fat. Now as I said not all fat is equal. We need healthy fat to help facilitate our circulation, reduce triglycerides (chemical fat stored in the body), and for proper brain development and functioning. We can obtain these benefits from healthy fats by consuming unsaturated omega 3 and 6 fatty acids. Unsaturated means its lipid at room temperature which makes it easier for our body to utilize. More specifically omega 3 and 6 fat acids are considered "healthy fats". We get omega 3's from sea food primarily and omega 6's from nuts and seeds obviously our incarcerated access to these types of fats are limited to tuna, sardine, and mackerel packs for 3's and peanuts, almonds, and cashew packs for 6's. In the world for convenience many of these fats are sold as oils made for cooking so that you can easily get your daily fat allowance. Unfortunately, we don't have access to those oils so for that reason "look to the packs". Read your labels on your store to severely limit anything saturated or partially hydrogenated e.g. honeybuns, donuts, little Debbie snacks, pastries and peanut butter. These are foods that will put on unwanted fat and cause you to feel tired, lethargic, and lacking in energy while at the same time having negative effects on your health.

Finally, at the risk of sounding redundant, nor are all carbohydrates created equal. They are named as such because chemically they are made up of sugars made out of carbons attached to water (carbo-hydrate). Carbohydrates are the preferred energy source of the body and the only energy source of the brain and red blood cells. In addition to being a key energy source they also stimulate the metabolism to utilize proteins for, muscle repair in a system called protein synthesis. One might assume that a bulking cycle would have higher protein and lower carbs than a cutting cycle but that is not the case.

A dirty bulk (or even a lean bulk) can call for 1-2 grams of carbs per pound of body weight and 8-1 gram of protein per pound. Whereas a cut diet can call for 8-1 gram of cabs per pound. As you can see an increase carbohydrates are the primary factor in mass gaining and likewise careful carb limiting and monitoring is the key to cutting. The other important component is what kind of carbs and at what times they should be consumed. This brings us to the difference between simple and complex carbohydrates. Now I'm sure everyone has heard about these complex carbs, but what are they really? I've posed this question to inmates and head everything from what bred to oatmeal to T-bone steak, to you name it. We've already discussed that carbohydrates are basically sugars. A carbohydrate is determined simple or complex by the rate at which it is broken down into glucose in the blood stream. We gauge this by rating different 1-100 that measures the rate and amount of glucose released into the blood stream over a 4-hour period. A 100 on the glycemic index would be equal to eating straight glucose and a 1 rating (which I wouldn't even be able to give an example of off the top of my head) would take the full 4 hours to release a minimal amount

Of glucose into the blood stream. Traditionally anything under a 70-gram rating would be considered a complex carbohydrate and anything over 80 will be simple with the middle ground being kind of ambiguous no man's land between simple and complex.

There are books out there that have exhaustive charts of the GI ratings of tons of foods or if you write of call family of friends that have 10 seconds and internet connection they can Google search "insert food name" GI rating. Some examples of complex carbs are brown rice, sweet potatoes, oranges, apples, whole grains, and whole grain cereals. Notice I said whole grains and not wheat bread because is really just enriched, processed, and food colored white bread which is definitely a simple carbohydrate. Other examples of simple carbs are white rice, regular potatoes, bananas, canned fruits, instant oatmeal, and of course ramen rice soups. Let me paint a picture of these simple carbohydrates for you. Let's take white bread. White bread was created out of necessity during the civil war period in the American south. When the troops were marching on long campaigns they would bring along whole grain flour for food. Often times the troops would find their flour infested with maggots that were drawn to the abundance of nutrients found in the flour.

Well us ingenuities southerners decided to bleach the flour removing all nutrients along with the maggot problem that came with it. Now the soldiers had maggot free food for their belly that had been completely stripped of the nutrients it had before. After the war it grew in popularity and became an American tradition still around today. Americans preferring unhealthy food over healthy food, now that's the America I know!

One last thing I want to touch on before moving to why we even came about the difference between simple and complex carbs is why I listed oatmeal amongst the simple carbs seeing as pretty much every jail in America has access to oatmeal. Steel cut oats and rolled oats (usually the ones that take 20-30 minutes to cook) are in fact complex carbohydrates and some of the best you can eat at that. Instant oatmeal (usually all we have access to at the store window) rate as high as a 90 on the GI putting them in the simple carb category. I had not previously realized this before my incarceration now I know why dropping below 8% body fat was always so difficult for me. I ate instant oatmeal every day and at the wrong time to consume a simple carb. So go easy on the oatmeal from the store window because it's not the complex carb we might assume all oatmeal is.

To better understand why knowing which kind of carbohydrates to eat at what time is important allow me to discuss the phenomenon of the "sugar crash". Everyone's experienced this whether on a free world birthday or an incarcerated holiday celebrated with a duplex cookie and honey bun cake. We feel our energy levels soar, maybe we get extra chatty at the spades and dominos table, we may even begin to sweat a little, or as what happened to me once after a piece of particularly rich Christmas cake our muscles may begin to tremble or spasm. This is all due to the metabolic response of eating simple carbohydrates. Our bodies suddenly have a lot of extra caloric energy on hand that our body is looking for an outlet for. Hence the metabolic response of having extra energy and the mental response of feeling jittery or amped up. If we don't use this extra energy (some research shows in a 30-60-minute window) than the body converts these extra carbs to storage or fat. The process of converting the extra carbs to storage or fat. The process of converting the extra carbs to storage through the digestive process can leave us feeling groggy and lethargic after the "sugar high" later resulting in the crush. To avoid such high and lows in the metabolic effect of carbohydrate consumption complex carbohydrates can be substituted for the simple ones. These carbs allow your body to have a steady supply of glucose over a longer periods of time. This leads too better and more prolonged feeling of fullness and helps your body keep from getting hungry again 2 hours after eating a ramen noodle soup or 30 minutes after eating a honey bun. A diet of only simple carbohydrates is like living in a house with a shoddy electric system. Sometimes the lights flicker, surge, dim, and go dark for extended periods. Likewise, a diet blended with complex carbohydrates is like paying that bill on time and getting strong, steady, electricity all day long. Now notice I said blended worth complex carbs. Obviously very few diets are feasible to eliminate all simple carbs. Especially incarcerated. Seeing as we are at a severe disadvantage with complex carb availability a lot of our task will be consuming complex carbs when we don't need them (there is no reason to eat a big ole piece of cornbread 3 times a day), and most importantly timing the simple carbohydrates we eat to maximum effectiveness.

So at least I bring you to the biggest weapon, aside from knowledge, in your jail hose nutritional arsenal. Timing. A was to avoid that sugar crush and put those excess simple carbs to use is to do just that, use them. In my younger years I had a trainer and he used to advocate something called a 30-30-30 rule; 30 minutes prior to training eat 30 grams of simple carbs and 30 grams of fast digesting protein. This gives you a spike of readily accessible carbs to use as energy for your workout and readily accessible protein to rebuild muscle tissue as you're tearing it down. Now you can make that white bread and kid's meal spaghetti dish work towards your advantage. Even more important than your pre-workout meal is your post-workout meal. For the hour after you work out your body is primed and ready to take in nutrients in a state called anabolic window. Anabolic means taking simple tissues or molecules and making them into more complex tissues proteins – Muscle tissue. Catabolism is taking more complex tissue and turning it into simple tissue or molecules, glycogen –glucose-ATP which is taking stored energy to actual energy. When consuming carbs and protein before your workout you decrease the catabolic accessible fuel and cell building blocks. Now in your 60-minute anabolic window after your workout. By consuming simple carbs during this anabolic window your body is able to more rapidly get the glucose back in your muscle that was expanded during your workout. In addition, the faster absorption rate of those carbs post workout will also maximally stimulate your body's ability to synthesis proteins during this precious anabolic window. Some research shows that not utilizing this window can inhibit muscular gins at a rate of up to 50%. That's a big difference. So if they won't feed us healthful complex carbs the next best thing is to time our simple carbs intake around our workouts and try to forego these simple carbs throughout the rest of the day. We can do this by saving the white bread off our lunch trays waiting till mid-afternoon to eat it, workout all the way till last chow, and eat all the cornbread and protein we can get our hands on during our anabolic window. For those inmates that simply feel like you have to eat at night save something simple from your late chow tray, eat it 30 minutes before your workout in the evening and then eat rice, beans, and protein as soon as you can after tour workout. When I do this I have my food cooking while am in the shower to be ready as soon as I'm out 30 minutes after my workout. With the late night meal try to still eat it at least 4 hours before you go to sleep so your body hormones have enough time to rebalance before bed.

These strategies are important for my weight-loss oriented guys but another one that some research has proven effective and that I definitely believe is effective from personal experience is doing cardio in a "carb-fasted-state", your body is in a carb fasted state when it has gone at least 10 hours without carbohydrates. Remember your body uses its energy in the order of carbs than fats, then proteins. If your body does not have any readily Accessible carbohydrates, then it will begin to utilize fat as its primary energy source. This can be achieved be doing cardio as soon as you wake up and then eating your breakfast right after your cardio session. I've made this happen by bringing a bowl to breakfast to save the meal until after I can set out to early rec I've adjusted my schedule to sleep all morning and turn lunch into breakfast after my cardio session. This allows my late night meal not to be such a late night meal as I stay up later. I've also just made my own breakfast of milk, oatmeal, and peanut butter so I can sleep through breakfast but not skip it. This carb-fasted cardio strategy has done wonders for me by stimulating my metabolism at the jump start of my day. This allows me to utilize the nutrients I consume throughout the rest of the day.

The last important aspect of timing is post-workout protein. I know I have emphasized a high simple carb and protein meal within 60 minutes of finishing your workout but eating a high protein snack ASAP will also benefit your gains. In the county we had protein bars, in prison we have protein snacks, and when my store account was low I saved milk from my breakfast trays and would have 2 milks with 2 oat meal packs to sit together during my workout. By the time I was done I had a delicious poor man's protein shake.

Now to sum up in one word what we can do to put this nutrition information into action would be practicing "discernment". The Bible has a lot to say on this topic that will help enlighten us on why it is important to be discerning. Let's go to Hebrew 5: 11-14 where the Bible even a food analogy to discuss the importance of practicing discernment. It reads "About this we have much to say and it is hard to explain since you have become dull of heaving. For though by this time you ought to be teachers, you need someone to teach you again the basic principles of the oracles of God. You need with not solid food, for everyone who lives on milk is unskilled in the word of righteousness since he is a child. But solid food is for the mature, for those who have their powers of discernment trained by constant practice to distinguish good from evil" Alright, many of us may have started a workout program in the past and neglecting to practice good nutrition we saw minimal results. Even though, by the amount of time we had been working out, our bodies should have been a testament to our success. Instead many of us stayed at beginner levels because we failed to discern what we should be eating. Our level of fitness called for us to be on "meat" (a healthful diet plan) but instead we continued to live on "milk" (eating sloppy, what we want, when we want. The Bible is saying that for our spirits to grow and mature (the Greek word for mature can also be "to make perfect") we must from God right now. If we fail to practice the discernment from good and evil. If we fail to practice the discernment from good and evil. If we fail to grow and mature our spirits. We may find ourselves, even as Christian men, set aside from the assignment, and blessings God has for our lives. Look at where we're sitting right now. I failed to discern good from evil and I was disqualified for a time, from the blessings of God until I had time to learn the "basic principles of God" and was given time to "practice to distinguish good from evil" and now I feel the blessing and assignment of God every day, even from a jail cell. This is how great our God is in 1 John 3:20-21. It reads "For whenever our heart condemns us, God is greater than our heart and he knows everything. Beloved if our heart does not condemn us we have confidence before God". In the physical, when we mess up our diet plans, it's easy to get discouraged and want to give up. What we have to remember is that God has given us amazing bodies that can overcome any bad eating habits we may have had or present nutritional slip ups we may have made. God is telling us that if we make a bad discernment or choice and that choice is discouraging us to the point we want to regress back to a lifestyle of bad choices, to take heart. God is bigger than our guilt, discouragement, and shame. Bring it to him, accept His forgiveness and leave it with Him. Another name for Satan is "The Accuser". He Wants to keep you from being blessed and used by God. Don't let him! Take your bad choice to God, He already knows what's up, and get back on track it is our reward for maintaining that "constant practice [of] discerning good from evil". In the physical it's seeing our waist lines shrink and our biceps bulge. Its feeling like you have energy to meet the day without feeling bloated, tired, and lethargic. In the spirit it's the satisfying feeling of knowing God is using you. It's the ability to stand boldly before the throne of grace and know your prayers are being heard because 1 Peter 3:12 says "For the eyes of the Lord are on the righteous and his ears are open to our prayers. But, the face of the Lord is against those who do evil"

Section 4

"Accountability"

"Accountability"

Alright men, today we're going to talk about how a little accountability can go a long way with helping us achieve our goals. Similarly, we are also going to discuss how important it is to choose the right partner.

How many of us have woken up on any given Tuesday and knowing its leg Tuesday, psyched our self-up for the mother of all workouts, only to have the brake thrown on us by our workout partner? "Bro I'm not really feeling it today...""" can't we just do pushups today?", or my favorite "my girl isn't answering the phone and I'm really not in the mood." If your girls not answering the phone you need to do something to relieve your stress and take your mind from the point of obsession son! If you've been working out while incarcerated, chances are good you've been on at least one side of that motivational (or lack thereof) fence. If this becomes a trend and you discover your workout partner really isn't "about that life "then it's going to be important to move on to someone that can match your level of motivation. Now I'm not saying that you should dump your workout partner the first time he's sick or needs a little encouragement to get up and go. I'm talking about the ones that you see around the pod all day until its "that time", you know what time we workout bro why are you in your rack? You said 30 more minutes 30 minutes ago. These are the ones that got to go. The Bible says in I Corinthians 15:33 Bad company corrupts good character." Not to say in this particular situation the partner that got to go is bad. Simply that bad workout habits can corrupt good ones. Plus, practically speaking, the workouts laid out in the programming chapter, by necessity, need a dedicated partner to provide resistance to help overload your muscles. There is nothing worse than being all decked up on coffee, rip, roaring, and ready to go, only to discover your weight has bailed on you today. By hard won experience I can tell you make sure you get a verbal commitment from your partner of the time and type of workout before getting all tweaked out on a bunch of coffee. And don't feel like you're being harsh by dumping your unmotivated partner. There is precedence for this in the Bible in I Corinthians 5: 1 - 5. This passage talks about a man caught up in sexual immorality and Paul commands the church to " turn over to satan for the destruction of his flesh, so that his spirit may be saved on the day of the Lord. " Paul realizes that the man is not going to change his ways only by external influences (i.e. the church). That change is going to have to come from within and what better way than by having to suffer some consequences for his actions. This is the difference between the partner needing a little bit of encouragement and the one whose heart just isn't in it. The difference between "iron sharpening iron "or" bad company corrupting ".

For an example of Iron Sharpening Iron, I give you from my experience, Paul. I had been in county for 3 months and my original partner had caught chain, so I was on the market. Paul was your average white collar criminal standing all of 5'7. I had peeped him out on the rec yard doing some squats and lounges. He tells me a few more weeks and he'll start working out with me. I tell him "great, just let me know ". In my head I'm thinking yeah I hear what you say but I believe what you do, well sure enough 2 weeks later Paul turns out for legs day, not only keeping up the with an entire routine that leaves me winded and makes 9 out of 10 people quit. Paul had the audacity to ask for more! Wow, that will teach me to ever make assumptions prior to investigation when it comes to what a determined person can do.

Let's take the example with Paul a step further talking about Iron Sharpening Iron. I came to jail thinking I was only going to be here for a day when after a rescheduled court date, a week later I got molly - whopped with 10 years. I'm not going to say I was mad at God, but I definitely was dealing with some self-pity and lack of spiritual motivation. Well, Paul was a Christian who had earned my respect through his drive and dedication to working out, especially being 20 years my senior. When he suggested a system for daily Bible study, I listened. 3 months after we'd began working out he suggested I read 3 chapters of the Old Testament everybody and pick a small section of the New Testament to re - read everybody for 15 days before moving on to a new section of the New Testament. Guys I still use this system today and my spiritual life has grown exponentially as a result. You may be asking yourself why I'm sharing this story with you. The reason is if you're reading this book people are most likely going to notice you know what you're doing. A few of them might ask you to workout with them. You now have the opportunity to be a "Paul" in that man's life. 9 times out of 10 your workout partner will turn out to be your closest friend in the tank/ pod/ unit you're at. If you know what you're doing and/ or have an unusual amount of drive/ determination that man may just look up to you. God has just given you an opportunity to help "spot that man's spirit ". Maybe you share what God's been doing in your life. Maybe you ask him what he learned in the world today, perhaps you offer Godly advice on his struggles. Say your partner isn't a Christian and you don't want to be pushy, but you still want to minister to him. Use that respect you've earned through your work out game and lead an example with your life outside work out time. Read the Bible out in the open so you can answer any spiritual question someone approaches you with. Try not to grumble when the CO's put you down but maintain a positive attitude. This will go a long way towards making people wonder about what sets you apart. Especially those whose respect you've already earned. God's plan for everyone isn't sending everyone to Africa as a missionary. General population in a jail or prison is one of the few places in the world missionaries can't just be sent. But if you're looking for ways to serve God, then start with the people that he's already put into your life.

There are two bodies of water over in the Middle East. The Sea of Galilee and Dead Sea. It is known that the Sea of Galilee has one of the richest aquatic eco - systems on the planet. Fishing is a huge part of life in the area because of overly abundant fish and vegetation found in that body of water. Now the Dead Sea is a different story as you may have surmised from the name. It's filled with salt and life is next to non - existent in this body of water. Two different bodies of water in roughly the same area, not too distant from each other, but as different as night and day in turns of life found in each. Why? The answer is that fresh water flows into the Sea of Galilee and flows out. We serve a God that tells us what he means and shows us. No matter how much determination and knowledge we think we have, if we're not using that knowledge and determination to encourage another and likewise not allowing someone else knowledge and determination to encourage us, it will be us that suffers in the long run. There are endless inmates out there that want to spend their time strengthening their bodies but might not know how. It's almost impossible to coach someone with good workout knowledge and ethics and then not practice them yourself.

You never know when God may be putting a Paul in your life saying "what next?". It's important to remain teachable and humble in the areas you need to and God can use anyone for that purpose. We just have to keep spiritual eyes open.

Alright now let's talk specifically about accountability. If any of you men have ever been to a free world gym what do you see on the walls? Mirrors! Those mirrors allow you to make sure your back is properly arched and you're going all the way down. Those same mirrors can also be used to make shanks and because most prisons are trying to limit the amount of shanks, chances are there are no mirrors where you're getting your work out on. This is where your workout partner comes in. There is no shame in having your form corrected, even if you've learned the proper form in the past. Your partner can see things that you can't see. Even the best of us revert to bad form sometimes when we're fatigued, our head isn't in it or perhaps we're trying something new.   Even Peter, the leader of the 12 disciples was corrected by Paul who wasn't even a part of the prestigious 12. If you check out Galatians 2: 11- 14 you find Paul reporting that he "Saw their conduct was not in step with the truth of the Gospel, I said to Peter." and then he "rebuked "or sternly corrected Peter. The Bible also tells us in Proverbs 27: 5 that "Better is open rebuke than hidden love ". We can learn a little lesson from our workout partner correcting our form that maybe we can apply to our brother spending a little too much time at the gambling table of looking at a magazine for the sole purpose of lusting after the women in its pages. Maybe you encourage each other to swear less or participate in positive conversations. Just being responsible for your partners physical well - being and not encouraging his spirit is, I believe, a big injustice. Let's not be afraid to step out of our comfort zones, like we do every day for our brutal workouts, to also build up our spirits and the spirits of those around us.

The last thing I want to talk about are the size of your workout crews. Again people are going to peep game and see you know what you are doing. You may have your crew of 1 or 2 others established and people will be trying to jump in. Learn how to set some boundaries in this respect. I never workout with more than 2 - 3 others so that you don't spend too much time in - between sets. Plus, put 4 dudes together when at most 2 of them are working out at the same time, the other 2 - 3 tend to get distracted. Plus, I know a lot of times the CO's might try to shut the workout down and big numbers draw heat.   Now by no means am I suggesting being rude and turning the man away with simply saying " sorry bro ". No explain to him the reasons above then brace yourself, offer to train him at another point during the day. We've got nothing but time and how do you think it'll look to that man if you sacrifice your time to help him. John 13: 13 says "Greater love has no one than this, that someone lay down his life for his friends." Laying down your life can be as simple as giving someone your time. Now you have the opportunity to be a Paul in yet another man's life. I can honestly say that the best times I've had incarcerated are the times I've helped someone else with serving God in mind. That is one of the great mysteries of being a servant of God, the blessings and satisfaction that comes from serving others. I hope this message helps you to seize that blessing for yourself. After all, don't take my word for it. Do the research for yourselves!

Section 5
CARDIO COMMITMENT

CARDIO COMMITMENT

Hey you'll today we're going to talk about everyone's favorite type of exercises, cardio! Now hold up muscle heads, before you tear this up and wait for next week's entry. Cardio helps you to get big, it is vital to maximizing your potential gains. But Big Steve's, Cardio for losing weight, how are you going to tell me it will help me build? Before we get into all that let's start with the basics.

Cardio is the Latin word for heart. You may picture running, jumping jacks, or burpees when you hear the word cardio. That is because these exercises are of a low intensity nature allowing the body to derive its energy from cell respiration which is the aerobic pathway for ATP or energy production. This is made possible by the heart taking in deoxygenated blood from the veins, oxygenizing it with air from the lungs and then delivering to the muscles as needed when exercise begins the concentration of blood in the body shifts from organs to the muscles. At rest the muscles contain about 15 - 20 % of your total blood. When exercises begin the muscles may contain up to 85 % of your total blood. That's a lot of blood. And I always wondered why thinking was so hard during wind sprints. It's because the vesting blood % in your brain is 15 % which drops to 5 % during exercise. But I digress, the point is that the heart is responsible for increasing the rate at which the blood is shunted out to the muscles.

<u>MUSCLE</u> and like any other muscle it needs to be strengthened and conditional for good fitness. Not only is that blood necessary for cardio, it is also responsible for delivering nutrients and flushing toxins from the muscles. I know most of you reading this are

familiar with that good burn you get while doing a set. What do you think makes that burn dissipate? The burn is from lactate build up which is a by - product of the anaerobic (without oxygen) process the muscles use to produce energy. Your heart pumping blood is what removes the burn allowing you to do your next set. Most of you also know that "pump "you get from a good workout. That pump is the blood your heart sends to the muscle being worked allowing it to maximize its effectiveness. The more blood, the rise force, equals move gain. The amount of blood being pumped in one heart beat is called your stroke volume. Stroke volume is a highly trainable factor allowing you to deliver more blood, oxygen, and nutrients with each beat.

Those are the performance advantages but the other major advantage is in the recovery. Most of us know that when we are working out we are breaking down our muscles with micro tears that tells the body they need to be rebuilt bigger and stronger. With anything in life before you build something you must first have the materials? Blood is the means of delivery. At rest your pumping approx. 1.5 gallons of blood a minute. During exercise this can be increased up to 5 - 10 gallons of blood a minute depending on your fitness level. That is a- board of nutrients for your muscles allowing yourself to build. faster and stronger. Please don't allow yourself to believe the myth that doing cardio is only for losing weight. I hope I've convinced you by now that that is simply not true.

One more myth I want to bust before suggesting programming is that steady state cardio is better at burning fat then high intensity interval training (H.I.I.T). It is true that steady state gets more of the calories used from fat, speaking percentage wise. The misconception comes in when someone fails to recognize the total calories being burned. A 30-minute exercise of a mph walk compared to a mph run, the walk burns a higher fat percentage but for few calories. Therefore, an exercise burning 240 calories with 40% from fat burns as fat calories. A high intensity exercised lasting the same 30 minutes (the run) burns 450 calories with only 25% coming from fat, burns 110 fat calories. Thus high intensity training does burn more fat even at the lower percentage. If you are able to train at high intensity don't let someone lead you off the path. Treat your cardio days with the same intensity as your push up days so that you can say you left your all on that rec yard.

But Big Steve, you said this entry wasn't about burning fat. Your right and that brings back to your heart being a muscle. I got on to my rep riders in my first entry because their lack of overload was severely limiting their potential for gains. It's the same way with your cardio. There is some benefit in steady state, but for really strengthening your heart and achieving benefits previously discussed, you need to push yourselves the same way you push your muscles, to overload. Any real gym rat knows you won't set big reppin 135 over and over and over again, you also won't maximize the effectiveness of your heart simply jogging 5 mph for 30 - 60 minutes. If you check last week's entry I have 2 workout programs for cardio. Both of them entail a warm up, working sets followed by recovery sets, with a cool down at the end. Your warm up should be about 10 - 15 minutes whatever the exercise, jogging or jumping jacks, etc., a good place to start the intervals would be 15 seconds at 90% of your absolute all followed by a 60 second recovery period, (50 % of absolute all). Start with 10 sets and work up to 15 sets as you progress. Once you hit 15 sets bump back down to 10 sets but up the intense intervals to 30 seconds followed by 60 seconds rest. Progress to 15 sets, bump back to 10 sets, up the intervals to 45, work up to 15, bump back to 10 sets and increase to 60 seconds. Progress to 15 sets and maintain. Remember this is now an anaerobic exercise just like resistance training because you are using more energy than oxygen in your blood alone can produce. Nevertheless, your heart will adapt to the specialized training to help provide as much energy as possible. This adaptation will only come through the process of it being overloaded, for the same reason long bouts of cardio will not be necessary. If you've been adding along with me, you're working sets will only take 30 minutes when you are fully conditioned and 12.5 starting out. If it takes you years to get the maintenance level that is fine. Do intervals twice a week and you will optimize your muscles potential, decrease recovery time, allow more food for your muscles, of course burn fat, increase your total metabolic rate allowing food you eat to be more effectively utilized, and lastly you just feel better. Your body releases loads of endorphins and hormones to meet the stress put on the body. The side effect is less over all stress and who among us doesn't need less stress! I hope I've convinced you to make some time and get sprinting.

Speaking of heart, Proverbs 4:23 says "keep your heart with all vigilance for from it flow the springs of life ". We've discussed how this is true in the physical but let's kick it up a notch and talk spiritual. The Hebrew word for heart meant more than the blood pumping oxygen. It was an ultimate word for the combination center of our very brains. Remember I Samuel 16:7 says "for the Lord sees not as men sees; man looks on the outward appearance, but the Lord looks at the heart." The heart is what concerns God.

He wants to know that our hearts are set on him and if they aren't then he wants to get us there. <u>MYTH</u>: God will never give you more than you can bear. The scripture I Corinthians 10: 13 says that he will not allow us to be tempted beyond our ability. But how does he develop in us the ability? By giving us more than we can bear. Just like the heart in interval training being overloaded and having to rely on the anaerobic process for energy. God will overload our flesh and have us rely on his process. The more he does this the stronger we grow. Many of us, especially in our positions, have asked the question how am I ever going to get through this? I'm not enough to go on. 2 Corinthians 12:9 says "My grace is sufficient for you for my power is made perfect in weakness". Our weakness causes us to rely on his power and not our own. For my brothers in Christ out there that are at the end of their rope, know that God is trying to build you up and make you stronger. Many of us may have just been running in Circes our whole life relying on our energy worrying about our own plans. Consider my brothers that perhaps God has a better plan for, but to give you the strength you need to accomplish them you might need to be trained in a way that is detestable to you. When I started doing intervals my only thoughts were "don't throw up" and "when will this be over", but when it was finally over the feeling was incomparable. Over time my heart became stronger and the effect it took to reach that same feeling was less. There is no maybe, God is preparing you for that feeling of peace from a heart set on him. He is preparing you for a purpose, for an eternal weight of glory beyond all comprehension. The only question is which way will you run? Towards him or away from him. My boy Jonah tried to run away, check out how that turned out for him

Section 6

Hormone Help

Hormone Help: Our body's chemical messages.

What's up men, today we are going to talk about hormones and how they can benefit us. Let's start out with a simple definition of what a hormone is. Hormones are chemical messenger's product inside the body that tell the body's organs to perform various functions. Examples of these hormones are testosterone, estrogen, growth hormone, insulin, and cortisol to name a few. These hormones can be safely manipulated to allow us to increase our gains, burn fats, and maximize our energy output for every workout. Testosterone and growth hormone are our main muscle building hormones. They respond to the body's need for mote help caused by overload, resulting in greater protein synthesis for greater gains. Growth hormone has the added advantage of being the #1 fat burner our body produces. We produce the most GH at the start of our workout and when we sleep. I will get to the sleeping part later but for now let's get started with how Testosterone, Growth hormone, and Cortisol affect our workouts.

Alright now, when our workout begins, one of the physiologic responses our body has is to increase the level of testosterone, Growth hormone, and Cortisol. These levels stay at a maximum working peak for 45 - 60 minutes. After 45 - 60 minutes' testosterone and growth hormone levels sharply decrease whereas cortisol remains high until you quit exercising. For this 2 reason, high - intensity workouts taking no longer than 45 - 60 minutes excluding warm up and cool down, are optional for maximum available function. Cortisol is a stress hormone. When the body begins its workout it undergoes a period of stress. The purpose of this hormone can be traced back to Paleolithic period where a cave man might go days without finding game for food. When he did kill game, cortisol will send the body messages saying it might be a while before it ate again and for that reason fat will be stored to help the caveman get through the stressful period until his next kill. Once your testosterone and growth hormone drop, continuing to work out will give you below average gains and encourage fat storage. Trust me; I was devastated when I learned this. I was a gym for 2 - 4 hours a day guy for years. My mood was terrible, my body fat wouldn't drop below 10%, and I felt like my chest gains were catastrophic. I answered it with working harder and longer which postponed the cycle. It wasn't until I was willing to learn and put into effect what I learned, that previous barriers could be shattered. Sometimes less is really more!

Now I know, I get it, we're all doing time, trying to bun time and that 3-hour w/o was a big part of our day. How can we get that back? I'm a very high energy individual and to maximize my workouts and still burn the maximum amounts of time I added cardio. Figure out what works for your routine whether it be 1000 jumping jacks or ten laps. Remember this is for my high energy guys or everyone with body fat they are trying to lose. Split your workouts with cardio in the morning & resistance at night or vice versa.

Now they're a few myths I would like to bust. The first of which is that if a woman lifts weights that she will put on bulky muscle. The truth is in the hormones. Females produce 1/16th the amount of testosterone as men. For that reason, it is virtually impossible for women to develop the bulky muscles they so greatly fear. That fear in addition is severely limiting many women from the metabolic and physiological benefits a simple resistance program would yield.

The second myth is the reason most people believe about eating carbs after 6 p.m. prevents weight loss. Notice I said "the reason ". The principle is still accurate that you should limit severally your carbs 4 hours before you go to sleep. The commonly believed reason is that your body won't be able to digest the carbs when you sleep so they will be turned into fat. This reasoning is false. When you ingest carbohydrates your body's blood sugar level will rise. Your body's response to this rise in blood sugar is increased insulin production that reduces blood sugar by converting it to glucose for energy or glycogen for storage. Research shows that while insulin production is increased, growth hormone production decreases. Remember from earlier that you produce the most growth hormone while you're asleep. If you

load up on carbs before bed, insulin
increases & your maximum potential growth
hormone production severely decreases. So
even though the reason why eating carbs
after 6 p.m. is a myth, the fact that you
shouldn't is a rock steady truth.
Unfortunately, I'll even take it one step
further. Not only are those late - night
carbs limiting your fat burning potential,
they are also limiting your protein synthesis
which translates to less musculature gain. I
know it's hard, especially being locked up.
Everyone wants to spread after last chow
but if we can learn some discipline in this
area we will see our gains increase
experimentally. I utilize peanuts, milk,
beans & sausage, & mackerel straight out of
the packet. No soups, no rice, no oatmeal,
those are all carbs. The only exception will
be if you have a late night workout. In that
case consume a post workout carb meal but
try to still leave a 2-hour window between

the meal & rack. After your workout your body is screaming for nutrients so your blood sugar levels should rebalance faster.

Alright now I feel like I would be remiss if I write about hormones & ignore steroids. We've all heard about them & many are curious about them, allow me to share a brief testimony with you. First off let's define them; steroids are synthetic hormones, pure and simple. They allow the body to heal, rebuild & use large amounts of nutrients from food for protein synthesis. For these sacrifices there are a hefty price including but not limited too balding, body hair growth, night sweats, increased blood pressure, emotional instability, anger, irritation & hostility. People on steroids can train for hours on end & have continual gains because of the elevated hormone rate in the body. This is a reason you need to be cautious getting your workouts out of body builder magazines. 95% of those guys are on steroids which mean the 40 - 60-minute rule goes out the window. They are doing artificially what we are doing naturally by keeping our workouts under 60 minutes & limiting carbs before bed. Guys, all the information aside, steroids are drugs. They are mind and mood altering substances. I buy & large revoked my probation by neglecting that fact. After 2 years of sobriety & dedication to fitness I was 6' 190 lbs. & 85% of. I was in the best shape of my life. I was also in the best spiritual condition of my life, volunteering at rehabs, going to school & balancing successful employment. I decide I want to take it to the next level and enter in the Europa body building contest in August of 2013. After careful & thorough research I planned & procured my steroid cycle & began New Year's Day. On January 5th 2013 I distinctly remember trying to hit my knees & pray & feeling utterly disconnected. That conscious contact with God I had cultivated was lost. Looking back, I realize it was because I had stepped into the realm of a living lie. I no longer trusted in the person that God made me to be. My love had shifted from being God focused to self-focused. Love gives & lust takes & I had crossed over from loving what God had blessed me with to lusting after that which I had not earned & did not deserve. The results were catastrophic. In a month I took up a night job bartending at a strip club, I began to have a road rage once a week. I was a terror to my loved ones, my one & love became the image I saw in the gym room mirror for 4 hours a day. My 2 years of hard work & progress disintegrated in three months, I pushed my body to the point of hernia. I had to withdraw from the competition for surgery. During my recovery I began drinking & a month later I failed my probation drug test for alcohol which resulted in my getting a 10-year prison sentence, so please don't walk out these gates & think that because most steroids don't show up on drug tests that you will be able to use them with impunity. Numbers 32:23 says "Beware your sins will find you out ". This is a biblical truth & it is inescapable. Many of you may be reading this & saying "my self-control is better than Big Steve's "I would never do those things ". I simply ask you that you look where you're sitting. Is a five inches to your biceps really worth the possibility of returning here? I pray that your answer is no & remains no.

Section 7

On the seventh day He rested

On the 7th day He rested

I know thus far we've primarily discussed
the art of work. Equally as important as
that work is the art of rest. Did you know
most of your gains occur while you are
sleeping? Of course you did because a few
chapters ago we discussed our natural
growth hormone levels are elevated while
sleeping. Now a plus side of our
incarceration is that we most likely have
plenty of time to sleep. Most research
shows adults need between 6-8 hours' sleep
every night.

This can easily be achieved but on the
other side of that token we need to be
careful not to oversleep 10+ hours a day as
this could result in our metabolism slowing
down. We also condition our bodies to tend
to stay in an anabolic state instead of
promoting a catabolic state through

developing healthy sleep patterns and remaining active while awake.

Another important reason to get adequate amounts of sleep is because it should help you resist snacking up on empty calories when you are tired your body is going to try to make up that lack of energy somehow. The next go to behind sleep is food of course. So if you're tired you might want to consider finding

Time for a nap instead of popping open a bag of flaming hot Cheetos! (Which I hope you're not eating, tired or not).

What about a day of rest from working out though do you really need it? The answer is an unequivocal yes. I've trained countless guys in jail, usually younger, who have a lot of aggression, stress, and hostility that they want to focus into a workout every day. A few times I've caught my partners asking what we are doing on rest day. When I tell them we've been going six days strong, we just did heavy chest yesterday, its rest day today. I'll turn around 30 minutes later to see them doing pushups out on the rec yard. While the effort and ambition is admirable and I definitely understand needing to take some negativity and focusing it into something positive, this doesn't negate the fat that our bodies need a day off. Neglecting this day, a week off can lead to a medical condition known as Overtraining. The symptoms include a heightened heart rate, slower metabolic rate, a suppression of appetite, reversal of your hard earned gains and the eventual breakdown of your muscle tissue and tendons past your body's normal scope of healthy repair.

Fellas I know we might have a lot of our plates emotionally anxiously waiting our sentencing, a deal from the DA, or dealing with a parole set off. Working out is a great way to deal with these stressors but it should not be out only way. If we are finding that we can't sit still and deal without a workout every day, then we need to take it to God in prayer. Exercise is a gift that God has given us, but it shouldn't be taken s more than that. Remember James 1:17 tells us "Every good gift and perfect gift is from above coming down from the father of lights". If we're viewing working out as the source of our stress relief instead of viewing it as a gift from Him who is the true source of out stress relief, then I fear we are missing the point entirely. The practical side is obvious; we rotate our muscle groups and take a day off to rest every week because that's the healthy way to grow. Now let's take it a step deeper and look at the spiritual side of this whole equation because remember we serve a God who uses physical examples to illustrate physical truths.

The people of Israel were Gods original chosen people. God used this nation to teach all people his promises ad commands. In Exodus 31:12 the Lord tells Moses to tell the people that "Above all you shall keep my Sabbaths, for this is a sign between me and you throughout your generations, that you may know that I, the Lord, sanctify you". Notice the words "Above All" that's because God was pretty familiar with human nature by now. He knew man left to his own self central devices would eventually implode upon himself. How easy it is for man to get swept away by greed, pride, and lust that He knew He had to institute a weekly, undistracted day of remembrance to remind His people who it is that truly "sets them apart" or sanctifies them. Remember, yes the day is important to God, but more important than the day is the concept behind the day. That all good and perfect gifts come from the father above. If we find ourselves so engrossed with our live that we find ourselves unable to sit back and spend time with our creator, then it might be time to ask ourselves what idol we've constructed standing in Gods proper place in our hearts.

Our idols can be our bodies, significant others, freedom, and a million, billion other things. God's solution to these idols was and still is to spend time with Him and reflect on the fact that I am God that sets us apart.

Looking back at my 3 relapses with a year + of sobriety I undoubtedly see the same formula. God keeps me sober and blesses me with a good job and just that quick I forget where those good gifts came from. God slowly gets phased out and the girlfriend, the perfect body, or just the good old simple arrogance that "I got this" begins to take Gods place. The old adage goes "Anything that you put before God you will eventually lose" Never have I returned back to destructive life styles when God had his proper place in my life. The best way to make sure He stays in that proper place is to spend time with him. In Ezekiel 20:23-24 the Lord says "moreover I swore to them in the wilderness that I would gather them among nations and disperse them through the countries, because they had not obeyed my rules but had rejected my statutes and profaned my Sabbaths and their eyes were set on their father's idols". Historically speaking the nation of Israel had no country and were spread among the nations from A.D. 70 – 1948, personally speaking I was uprooted from my home and shuffled through 15 units all across the state of Texas before finally landing at my ID camp. God can't lie, if He says the consequence for rejecting His rightful

place in our hearts is scattering and
dispersing us, He will bring it to pass.

Section 8

Something Outta Nothing

Alright men, I know I was letting my rep reads have it last week, but the fact is I got to give those boys their due. They're doing the best they can with the information they have, getting up, getting out, and getting something. How many of us have heard other inmates tell us "I'm going to wait until I get out before working out". Let me be clear about this, if you can't act right in here, your **MOST LIKELY** not going to act right out there. We have been blessed with the unique opportunity to be freed from our life of responsibilities and distractions (looking on the bright side here), so let's use it to develop as many health habits as possible. The purpose of this entry is to try to eliminate any excuse by helping you to make a well-rounded workout programmer without having a Gold's Gym membership. I spent 2 years in county dodging CO's and working out in the only place the camera couldn't see the bathroom, and the rec yard. After a fair amount of trial and error this is what I've come up with.

First off I want to stress the importance of knowing what you're going to do before you start your workout, going out there and free styling is not going to cut it ya'll! The reason being is it's easy to get distracted, as you get tired you may quit early, and finally I'll bet you have a workout partner or 2 or 3. If you haven't established what your workout for the day will look like it'll be like trying to lead 4 horses with 1 piece of rope.

Second, you CAN NOT do pushups every day and expect to see substantial gains. Muscles need a minimum of two days to recover and as many as 5 depending on the intensity of the workout. These will be moderate to intense workouts that will need the higher end of that result schedule

before you're ready to blast them again.
Remember, just because you're no longer
sore does not necessarily means your
muscle are done recovering. Soreness or
DOMS (Delayed Onset Muscle Soreness) is
an indicator of lactic acid build up which is
a by-product of the anaerobic process.
Just because your body has eliminated the
acid build up, or because you don't feel sore
to begin with, does not necessarily mean
your muscles are fully recovered. To keep
the beast mode workouts flowing, it will be
necessary to alternate muscle groups so
your muscle gets the rest it needs. Any
workout longer than 45-60 minutes is over
kill and I'll explain why in two weeks in an
entry called "Hormone Helpers". For now,
know my exercise programming will take 45-
60 minutes, with a target range of 15 sets,
consisting of 5-12 reps a set. So let's set
started

-

<u>*Monday-*</u>

Chest and shoulder start 10 minutes' light cardio warm up

<u>5 sets of 5-10 flat resistance pushups</u>- For this exercise you need your workout partner pressing down on your shoulder blades. He should be pressing hard enough where you fail before your 10th rep. keep pressure consistent, if you can find something to balance on your partner may even stand on your shoulder blades as your strength progresses. I like to take towels or laundry bags and wrap them around my hand between my knuckles and 2nd finger joint. This allows me to do the pushups on my knuckles mimicking holding a bench press bar. This will also allow your elbows to bend outwards putting the focus on your chest and off your triceps.

<u>5 sets of 5-12 dips</u> – I've used tables pushed together, chairs pushed together,

and adjacent bunks for an even level platform to perform the exercise. Plant arms at your ides not behind your back. If 12 reps become too easy up modify the exercise to hold up to 5 seconds at the bottom of your rep. Elbows bend to 90° angle to lower yourself down, then fully extend up.

5 sets of 5-12 body weight military presses or handstand pushups-

For hand stand pushups have your spotter assist your legs up into a handstand with back toward wall. Keep your gaze horizontal to help to help keep your spine straight. Allow your spotter help you balance as necessary. All but tap your head on the ground with every rep. for an easier modification, find a table, rail, or platform to put your toes on with hands planted on the ground. Make an "L" with your body so that the work is being done by your shoulders and not your chest. Use these to build your way up to handstand pushups. End 10-minute light cardio and stretching cool down.

The next muscle group will be legs. This is the biggest muscle group on your body guys. It is CRITICAL not to neglect them fellas. Now unfortunately it is very hard to achieve overload without a squat rack. I've experimented doing squats with another inmate on my shoulders but let's face it, no one likes sweaty gene Talia pressed up against their neck. For that reason, this legs day will start with an explosive superset and lead into a circuit compound set. Our legs are little different from our other muscles because they are used to carrying our weight all day long therefore we can push them harder than our upper body. For the lack of weight to increase the workouts intensity we will cut the sets down by combining them and eliminating over half of the rest periods. 3 super sets flowed by 3 compound sets. Sounds easy right? Alright here it is

Tuesday – Legs

<u>3 Sets of 6-12 box jumps SS with 3 sets of 10 each</u>

Find a knee to waist platform that is stable. Start on the ground in a deep squat position. Explode and jump upwards onto the platform to land in a deep squat position. Jump backwards and land on the ground in a deep squat position. This is one rep, be sure to and on our legs shoulder width apart and do not lock out your knees. Go immediately to the next exercises in the superset. To perform this, you need a good amount of room. Stand up straight. Drop into a lunge by crossing the right foot behind your planted left foot. Lightly tap right knee on the ground. Now explode up and sideways off your lift foot and land on your right foot. Try to clear 2-3 feet between the planting foot and the landing foot. Now plant the landing right foot and cross the left behind down into a lunge and lightly tap left knee. This is two reps 1 on each leg. Remember guys were doing explosive exercises first to prepare our legs for over load in the body weight compound circuit next.

3 Sets on the compound circuit: - Find a lane 15-20 feet if possible. One side to side diagram.

6-10 lunges down/ 10 jump scissor lunges/6-10 lunges home

6-10 squats down (face sideways and on toe after every rep) / 10 jump squats / 6-10 squares home

6 leap frogs down / 10 jump sumo squats/toes 10 and 2 legs shoulder width/ High knees back (baby steps)

While your partner is resting you are doing your set and vice versa

This workout is a beast and will only take 30 to 45 minutes so feel free to add core exercises like sit ups and leg throws at the end.

Once this workout becomes easier to you, you can up the intensity by making your squats and lunges double taps on the same rep before your progression

Wednesday-Back and Bicep

start 10 minutes' light cardio pull up

<u>5 Sets of 5-15 wide grip pull ups</u> – If these are easy for you it might just be that you are not going all the way down and all the way up. Have your partner watch your form? Don't be afraid to ask your spotter to grab your feet to help you up. It's better to have good form and a spot than to try to prove your manhood with bad form and get minimal gains. As a bar I have used the railing that holds bathroom stalls together. The "foot board railing of side by side bunk beds, a broom stick laid across non symmetrical top bunks, or a sheet tied between two anchor points. Get creative guys, I know we don't have a lot to work with but if you think outside the box am sure you can convert one out of what you get assuming you're not in the hole.

Your partner to pull your arms down so that you get the negative side of your rep and he gets some action working his back. Remember guys we're not trying to kill each other but make it challenging.

Thursday cardio -

Now some of you might be saying cardio? I don't need to lose weight; I just want to get big. Well guy's bad news, cardio is a crucial element to muscle growth and I'll explain why in -depth in a few words. Don't worry this won't take long. It's your choice whether you want to do the cardio or core first. I like core first so I wrote it in that order. It will also be near impossible to overload your core with resistance without weights so we'll do the best we can.

<u>3 Sets of 20-40 leg throws</u>- Hold your partner's ankles while you bring your straight legs up to his hands for him to throw in alternate directions.

<u>3 Sets of 20-40 Jack Knives</u>-Lay on our back and bring your straight arms and legs together over the mid-section of your body.

<u>3 Sets of 20 supermen's</u> – Lay on your stomach and raise straight legs and arms off the ground. Hold for 1 second at the top

<u>3 Sets of Isometric holds</u> – 10 leg lifts/ hold feet 6" off the ground, 10 seconds, 10 seconds of flutter kicks / 10 seconds of leg scissors / 10 seconds hold/ end – increase difficulty by putting hands on your chest and then increasing to 15 seconds

<u>Pick and Internal Cardio Routine</u>

Sprints- 25 laps steady pace [/10 sprints/ 5 slow recoveries laps/] repeat 5-10 times/ 25 laps steady state

The warm up 25 should take about 10 minutes, the sprints should take about 20 minutes, and the cooled down 25 should take about 10 minutes.

The sprints are ¼ distance of the laps. If one full circle is a lap sprint is running through the circle one way in a straight line

Indian Run-10 brisk pace laps followed immediately by 3 full out circle sprints. Do 10 sets like this

The difference between sprints is steady, fast, slow, steady, whereas the Indian run is brisk, fast, brisk, fast, brisk.

Sprints come out to 75 laps and 50 sprints

Indian run is 100 laps and 30 sprints.

You may now take a day off and repeat the cycle.

Feel free to modify and tweak this program as you see fit. Just try to stay in the set #'s and intensity parameters.

Other chest exercises I like to cycle in are dive border pushups, or skull crushers. There are tons of different xxx and push ups modifications. I'm also sure y'all have a lot of great ideas for ab exercises. Build the program that works for you but don't sell yourself short. Lastly don't run from legs and cardio, they're your friends and necessary to essentially everyone's fitness goals.

Every 90 days you should take a week off or just engage in light cardio. Allowing that rest will prevent over training and muscle breakdown and bring you back refreshed next week. If you're like me and have a lot of energy, feel free to stretch and do cardio.

Ok guys I think that's it on programming. None of the other ones should be like this but was essential to fully explain and lay out the groundwork for your house work out program.

My man the Apostle Paul wrote little more than half of the New Testament. We

have something in common with Paul. We've
all been prisoners, were all been humbled
and we've all had to do with out in
Philippians 4:12 he said "I know how to be
brought low, and I know how to abound. In
any and every circumstance, I have learned
the secret of facing plenty and hunger,
abundance and need." Let's face it, a lot of
us probably look at "getting out" as the
answer to all our problems, I know it's easy
for me to think that way. But the truth is
when we're out there with a full gym and
proper nutrition we are still going to face
the spiritual difficulties of life. There will
be times that it feels like we are in a
spiritual desert for no apparent reason.
There will be temptations to give up, go
back, and return to that old way of life all
the time. Our first line of defense will be
the contentment we've learned through our
incarceration with our being contentment
we've learned through our incarceration

with our being brought low. If we're grateful for what we have, we will be less likely to succumb to that temptation to lust after that which is not ours. God has given us the key in Paul's next verse". I can do all things through Christ that strengthens me". There is an old saying "where there is a will there is a way". The purified truth is that where there is Gods truth there is NO way anything can come on the way. We've been brought low fellas, working out in bathrooms, stopping mid workout for a head count, getting locked down foe having too many socks and getting" surprise" rest day. Let's use these lessons the good Lord is teaching us to "abound in every circumstance" inside and outside these walls.

Such a thing as a "New Testament Christian". God gave us the old to show us why we need the new. For those that proclaim that the law has been abolished let me point out that our Lord himself said in Matthew 5:17 "Do not think that I have come to abolish the law and the prophets, I have come not to abolish them but to fulfil them". There you have it from our Lords own mouth. The letter of the law being replaced with the intent of the law. It also says in Galatians 3:24 "so then, the Lord was our guardian until Christ came, in order that we may be justified by faith". Let me tie these two verses together by a quote from A.W.Tozer he said "you can't have Jesus as savior in your life if you don't have Him as Lord in your life as well". I believe this is the heart of the matter. We know from Acts that the Holy Spirit wasn't imparted unto us until Jesus Christ ascension. In the Old Testament times the "guardian" of the law was needed until the era of grace. Now that grace has come do we forget that God has "Set us apart"? By no means, instead, having been justified by faith, we allow Christ to rule supreme in our hearts which then crystalizes into a sanctified life allowing us to be the "Lights of this world" that God has called us to be. So brothers, remember, rejoice for this is the day that the Lord has made. Be glad.

Getting Big

Resting Metabolic Rate "Getting Big to lose weight"

Alright men, now I know a lot of my focus in these entry's thus far has been on strength training. Many of you out there may be saying that you don't really care about the size of your chest and your arms, and doing less seems like way more effort than its worth. Your goals may be more centered on weight loss and the strength training aspect has very little appeal to you. Well a few sections ago I explained to my strength oriented guys why cardio was necessary for their goals. Well gentlemen every coin has two sides so this entry will be geared towards educating my weight loss oriented guys how strength training is beneficial towards their goals as well.

Most of us have most likely heard at some point in our lives that muscle weighs more than fat. This is true because muscle is a more complex tissue than adipose or fat tissue. Seeing as muscle tissue or a person's "lean mass" is a more complex tissue it therefore takes more calories to maintain that tissue. This is one of the primary reasons that those of us who began our incarceration with a high percentage of lean mass lost a lot of it sitting around in county. Our calories required to maintain our muscle were more than our calories being consumed, so our muscle tissue was broken down to lower the daily need, as well as produce calories to cover the deficit. Those of us who began our incarceration with a high fat percentage and continued to gain fat can also attribute the fat gain to an excess of non-nutritious foods and an increased sedentary life style. From sitting in our cells, to sitting I our day room, to sleeping in our bunks it is probably safe to say that our daily activity levels decreased upon our incarceration. The less activity daily, the less calories burned daily. For this reason, the American Council of exercise has suggested that taking at least 7000 steps a day can significantly increase the body's metabolic rate on a daily basis. I know our rec time may be limited but I achieved this goal in county by reading a book and walking in a triangle where everyone of the 3 sides were 3.4 steps in length. I knew after an hour at a brisk clip I could hit the 7000 step target. Keep in mind that there are 3600 seconds in one hour. That means approximately two steps a second will allow you to reach this goal. The book helped me to break up the monitoring of this activity but, just because it is monotonous, don't allow it to hinder you from reaping the benefits of its effectiveness. We were created with activity in mind. Don't allow the unnatural state our governing authorities have imprisoned us in to be the end of our active lifestyles. A little bit of effort over a long period of time can have impressive results. Fortunately, most of us have a long period of time to achieve those results so let's get started today.

Back to muscle weighing more than fat. Many of you may be saying Big Steve my goal is to lose weight and not gain it by putting on undesired muscle weight. Why should I waste time strength training and especially why should I go through the pain and effort of training my legs?

Well let me start off by saying I'm here to tell you that developing that muscle is your best friend to shaving off unwanted pounds. Even though the additional muscle will cause an increase in body weight as lean mass increases, that increase will be severely offset by the heightened level of fat loss. For most people the amount of weight from muscle mass gained will compare in comparison to the amount of weight loss from body fat reduction. Let's crunch some numbers on this, The Mifflin.st.Jeor Equation (Frankzufield, Roth-Yousey, and Compher, 2005; Frankenfield et al, 2003; Mifflin et al.1990) states that in men RMR (Resting Metabolic Rate) = (9.99 x weight) + (6.25 x height) - (4.92 x age) – 161. So inputting my weight of 220 and my height of 6 translated into metric is 100kg and 180 cm and age of 25. This equation comes out to a RMR of 2016 for me individually, now his level of RMR can be increased up to 1.9 times solely based on my body composition and activity level resulting in a new RMR of a whopping 3830 calories per day. Now given that is the maximum allowable increase, and most likely won't be achievable unless we end up with an outside job entailing all strenuous activity. This is just to give you an idea of how big an effect our body composition and level of physical activity can have on the amount of calorie our bodies can use for energy before they are converted to fat for storage. After all that is the CMX of the weight loss issue. We have taken in more calories than our RMR tells us we can burn in the same day creating a calorie surplus. A daily need of 2000 calories accompanied by a 2500 intake creates a 500 calorie surplus. Research has proven that 3500 calories is equivalent to one-pound body weight therefore a 500 calorie surplus every day for a week will result in gaining 1 pound per week until the surplus is topped or the RMR is raised. For those of us trying to lose weight the process is exactly the opposite. Consume 1500 calories a day with RMR of 2000 and we will create a 500 calorie deficit resulting in us losing approximately 1 pound per week. The other alternative is to consume 2000 calories with a 2000 calorie RMR and then to exercise at a rigorous intensity for an hour burning the additional 500 calories to create the deficit. The final alternative is to increase you RMR through strength training which produces a higher amount of lean mass resulting in a higher RMR. Yes, weight loss can be essentially that simple. Now I've harped on the importance of especially training your legs and that reason is also simple. Your legs are the biggest muscle group in your body. By neglecting them you are severely limiting your potential maximum RMR. The other reason relates to the hormone chapter last week. Research has proven that serum testosterone and Growth hormone levels can be increased by training multi-joint compound exercises (i.e. Squats and deadlifts) at 85-9% of your one rep max or moderate to high volume training with multiple sets and exercises and less than 1-minute rest intervals (Kramer 1988). So since testosterone and growth hormone are the 2 major hormone for muscle development, and by developing our muscles we can increase RMR, then by training our legs to release these hormones, we increase our RMR dramatically over time. The legs day include in the workout programming period focus on high intensity-short rest internal exercise which will help you to increase testosterone levels, burn fat, and build muscle. Please utilise it and don't sell yourself short.

So we've been discussing the principle of RMR which can be simplified to our physical "daily need" of calories. Well just as we have our daily needs in the spiritual realm. When the people of Israel were in the wilderness God provided them Manna every day to eat. This scripture is the origin of the principle of "Our Daily Bread". In the New Testament Jesus has told us in John 6; 35 that "I and the bread of life, whoever comes to me shall not hunger, and whoever believes in me shall never thirst". For that reason, as important as those calories are for are physical health. Even more important is that Bread of Life for our spiritual health. That Bread consists of spending daily time in prayer and daily time in his scripture. There have been times where I have tried crazy diets that called for severe calorie deficits. While adhering to those I would find that I no longer had the energy to do my everyday tasks. Sometimes the deficit was so severe that my thought life was affected. Why should it be any different spiritually? It isn't fellas. When my spiritual bread is deficient my spiritual energy just isn't there. That daily bread allows me to approach spiritual matters "weight" with the word of my Lord going through my head. That spiritual bred encourages me and strengthens me to maintain a level of spiritual fitness that is simply impossible without it.

Now remember earlier we talked about our RMR increasing as we develop muscle and grow. The more developed our physical becomes; the more calories become required to maintain that physique. The word of God is like that as well. When I was a baby in Christ reading the word and praying seemed almost like a chore. I would spend a little time or do a good deed and call it a day. The amazing thing, as many of us have or will discover, is the more time we spend with Christ, will result in wanting to spend even more time with Christ. Our desire for his word begins to increase. Our desire to obey his commands begins to increase. Our desire to spend time with our spiritual family increases. All of this because we've grown spiritually. As we put that spiritual muscle I believe satan steps his game up. The devil doesn't like us being happy and joyful and living in God's blessing. He's going to start shooting those shots our way, but remember, God has provided us with a way to resist. One of those ways is by spending time with him and allowing him to mold and shape our spirits. Hebrews 5:11-14 says "About this we have much to say and it is hard to explain, since you have become dull of hearing. For though by this time you ought to be teachers, you need someone to tech you again the basic principles of the oracles of God. You need milk, not solid food for everyone who lives on milk is unskilled in the word of righteousness, since he is a child. But solid food is for the mature, for those who have their power of discernment trained by constant practice to distinguish good from evil. A lot of us may have been hearing the word for a long time, but our hearing was dull because we were unskilled in the works of righteousness. I like to call this being a spiritual sissy. Maybe we thought that we could get by with the bare minimum or none at all. That spiritual calorie deficit has kept us from being the leaders and priests that God has called us to be. The text says we should be teachers but instead we need to be taught again. We should be eating meat but because of our immaturity we're on that milk diet, but fear not brothers, the solution is in verse 14. It says that the meat is for the mature who have practiced distinguishing good from evil.

We get the knowledge of how to discern from the spirit of Christ. We grow in the spirit of Christ by spending time I his word and praying so we may discern good from evil and become skilled in the word of righteousness A.K.A being spiritually yoked. AS we mature and develop onto that meat diet it's because the Lord has blessed us with those spiritual gains. Now it's our job to get those spiritual calories up by discerning right from wrong. Get strong and stay strong brothers.

Peace to you all and God Bless You!

Personal Fitness Goals

Your Notes What will you do?